COMPUTERS
AND
VISUAL STRESS

How to Enhance Visual Comfort
While Using Computers

Edward C. Godnig, O.D.
and
John S. Hacunda

Seacoast Information Services, Inc.
Charlestown, Rhode Island

AAW 9884

COMPUTERS AND VISUAL STRESS
How to Enhance Visual Comfort While Using Computers

Cover Design & Illustrations: Gatie Associates
Printing and Binding: Chadis Printing Company

Printed in the United States of America

Library of Congress Catalog Card Number: 90-60621
International Standard Book Number: 0-9625708-5-0

ACKNOWLEDGEMENTS

Many individuals have been responsible for the completion of this book. First the authors wish to thank the members of their families for support and inspiration during the preparation of this book.

Special thanks to the following individuals for their invaluable assistance:

Reviewers:
John Bessette
Loren Coen, Ph.D.
Edward C. Godnig, Sr.
Carl F. Gruning, O.D
Peter Hacunda
David Oliveira
Lawrence Ritter, O.D.
Bradford D. Smith, O.D.
Benjamin B. Stone, Ph.D.
J. Baxter Swartwout, O.D.
David Townsend, Ph.D.
Deborah York

John Gatie - graphic design
John S. Hacunda, Sr. - printing consultant
Edward Raso - desktop publishing

TABLE OF CONTENTS

PREFACE

This book had its beginnings, like many other projects in life, with a problem. Several years ago, I began working with computers as a programmer. A great deal of my working time was spent focusing on a computer screen and I began to experience visual discomfort. The first year I used computers on a full time basis I noticed that my sight was not as clear. Indeed, an eye examination revealed that my vision had changed. I had become more nearsighted and now required a lens prescription for my left eye.

I continued to experience visual problems on the job. As a programmer, I often had to concentrate on code on the screen for long periods and was under pressure to meet job deadlines. In retrospect, I realize the computer workstations I used were not set up with my comfort in mind. I suffered in silence. I imagined the discomfort I experienced was the price to be paid for doing the job.

On a chance conversation with Dr. Godnig, I mentioned my problem and he suggested some actions I could take to reduce my eye discomfort. The advice was helpful, but lead to further questions about this high tech health concern. Unfortunately, I discovered that much of the information regarding computers and visual stress is contained in technical scientific reports. But there is a lack of concise sources of information directed at the general public. This discovery became the idea for this book.

Helping to write this book has been an educational experience. It is surprising to learn that there is considerable disagreement even among the "experts" about the link between computer use and eye problems. The area of health effects of computer use is one of intense debate these days. I am still learning and striving to keep up with the latest developments. I do know that I am now better informed, and can perform my work using computers with greater comfort.

John Hacunda
December, 1989

CHAPTER 1 - A HIGH TECH HEALTH CONCERN

Are you among the estimated 40 million Americans using video display terminals (VDTs) on a regular basis? If so, do you often experience difficulty focusing on distant objects after prolonged VDT use? Do you suffer from eyestrain, irritated eyes, headaches, or any intermittent blurring of images on the screen? Have you noticed any blurring of vision beyond close range?

These are among the most common complaints optometrists hear from individuals suffering visual difficulties while working with computers. Two common problems are eye focusing breakdown and eye coordination anomalies. Individuals whose focusing systems are somewhat fragile are usually able to cope with normal reading and writing tasks. However, with prolonged use of a VDT, subtle visual difficulties can become permanent problems.

In addition to the problems cited above, other symptoms of visual stress include: posture changes; neck, shoulder, and back pains; frequently losing your place while trying to concentrate on a work task; and excessive fatigue or irritability. Workers may show a general decline in productivity, including increased errors and reduced speed while performing a task.

DIRECT SIGNS AND SYMPTOMS OF VDT-INDUCED VISUAL STRESS

* Eyestrain
* Blurred vision
* Irritated or reddened eyes
* Headache during or after VDT use
* Eye focusing difficulties when shifting from screen to distance viewing
* Doubling of vision
* Color perception changes
* Difficulty concentrating on work tasks
* Symptoms persist even when wearing eyeglasses
* Present prescription glasses cause discomfort

INDIRECT SIGNS AND SYMPTOMS OF VDT-INDUCED VISUAL STRESS

* Neck or shoulder tension, pain
* Back pain
* Excessive fatigue when using VDT
* Irritability increases when using VDT
* Pain in arms, wrists, or shoulders when working on VDT
* Increased nervousness
* Lowered visual efficiency and more frequent errors

To understand why there is an ever increasing number of health complaints associated with computer use let's consider the condition of the typical worker in the United States. Over the last 200 years there has been a profound change in the our society's economy. When originally founded, the United States had an agriculturally based economy. In the early 1900s the US economy was transformed from farm to industrial. Beginning in the 1960s there has been a shift from an economy dependent on mass production to one which is becoming popularly known as an "information society." [1,2]

While the transition from a farming to an industrial society evolved over a 100 year period, the change from an industrial to information society occurred in only two decades. The development of microprocessor technology and the advent of the personal computer in the late 1970s paved the way for the growth of the information age. Whether we are talking about fields as diverse as banking, education, engineering, transportation, telecommunications, health, or law, the emphasis today is on creating, processing, and distributing information mainly by using computers. Computers have become so commonplace that even elementary school children use them to learn in the classroom or to play video games at home.

Paralleling the farm-industrial-information shift in the economy is an increased demand on the eyes for close-up work. For example, the airline reservation agent, data entry clerk, computer programmer, telephone operator, and word processor must focus on computer terminals at very close range. However, we must remember that our eyes are adapted for distant viewing.[3] Our ancestors depended on keen sight while hunting. Research indicates that human traits - vision included - are selected because of their survival value to the individual and the species as a whole. Nowadays, in our more literate society, the use of our eyes within arms length is becoming increasingly important.

The change in emphasis on our visual system from distance viewing to close-up viewing has occurred in less than 50 years. Our visual system is unable to handle this increased use of near vision naturally. Instead we must actively adapt by modifying our work environment and work behavior. Table 1 shows how preferred visual working distances have shifted with changes in the United States economic conditions.

TIME	ECONOMIC EVOLUTION	VIEWING DISTANCE AT WORK
pre-1600's	Hunter-Gatherer	Far
1600-1800's	Farmer	Far
1900's	Laborer	Varied
1960's	Clerk	Near
1980-1990's	Information Worker	Near

Table 1. Predominant Visual Working Conditions in the United States Region

Visual stress is a very real problem for many VDT users. A panel of vision experts assembled by the National Research Council found that in most surveys of occupational VDT users, more than 50% of the workers experienced visual discomfort.[4] In the United States there are an estimated 40 million people using VDTs. That number is expected to increase to 100 million workers by the year 2000. Add this to the number of information workers on a global basis and the numbers and potential problem become truly staggering.

Many of the existing studies on VDT-related health complaints suffer from poor research design. This makes it difficult to distinguish among factors related to VDT use from other characteristics of the work environment. The nature of VDT work, including such variables as job type, visual tasks required, and hours per day, make generalizations difficult. There is also difficulty with providing an objective measurement or definition of "visual fatigue" or "eyestrain." Many of the eye discomfort symptoms experienced by VDT users are similar to those reported by other workers who perform near-visual tasks (e.g., typists).[5] Because of this the academic and scientific communities have adopted a "wait and see" attitude about whether there is a causal link between VDT use and eye problems. The prevailing consensus maintains that there is nothing inherently damaging about using a VDT. This conclusion is based in part on the ambiguity that surrounds the present state of our knowledge.

Shortcomings from some of the early VDT findings are being replaced by more rigorous studies by the academic and research communities on VDT use and its effects on workers. This is an area of intense public interest and research results are currently being used to develop labor and legislative policy. Recent legislation (1989) submitted to the New York City Council proposes improved eye care and working conditions for employees using VDTs. The proposed legislation provides for free biannual eye examinations and eyeglasses for employees who use VDTs for 20 hours or more per week. Dr. Jesse Rosenthal, a professor at the State University of New York College of Optometry, gave expert testimony supporting this legislation, based in part on research findings at the College's Center for Vision Care Policy. The study found eyestrain symptoms among 91 percent of VDT operators, and a direct correlation between the severity of symptoms and hours per day of VDT use. However, among workers supplied with specially prescribed VDT eyeglasses, 94 percent noticed improved comfort and 82 percent reported better working efficiency.

Bob Dematteo, a Canadian labor representative, examines the treatment of the VDT issue in his book *Terminal Shock*.[6] He suggests that if history is any future predictor, then the proof of establishing workplace and environmental hazards often falls on the shoulders of the user and not the regulators. The track record for asbestos, ureaformaldehyde, DDT, DES, contraceptive pills, and thalidomide gives testimony to public health regulation formulated after the fact. The burgeoning interest in reported VDT-related health complaints will ultimately shift the focus of attention from a medical and technical problem to a political and economic problem.

While these issues are being resolved there is still much that can be done now to enhance the comfort of VDT users. Two approaches can help improve VDT working conditions. The first involves **ergonomics**, which is the study of how the work environment, including equipment design and work tasks, relates to the job performance of the human worker. The goal of ergonomics is to increase worker comfort, productivity, and safety. In the case of the VDT workstation there are many changes that can be made to improve worker comfort and efficiency. The second approach is an **optometric** one, which concentrates on improving visual skills. An individual with properly conditioned visual skills is better able to cope with the visual demands of the VDT working environment.

There is a branch of optometry, known as **behavioral optometry**, that takes a holistic approach towards improving vision. Vision is viewed as a complex process which includes learning, that can be altered and improved by following the proper regime. This holistic approach can encompass areas as diverse as visual training procedures, diet, work organization, and education, all with the goal of improving the visual comfort and efficiency of the individual.

The purpose of this book is to explore **visual stress**, an increasingly prevalent health concern resulting from the computer age. The book first outlines the visual stress problem and then provides information to help prevent it. The organization of the information in the book is as follows:

Chapter 2 presents background information on the functioning of both visual and computer systems.

Chapters 3 describes the visual stress problem in terms of symptoms and causative factors.

Chapter 4 gives suggestions on creating an ideal workstation environment.

Chapters 5 provides information on an optometric approach towards reducing visual stress. The chapter covers the following subjects:

- key visual skills needed for VDT viewing
- requirements of a proper eye examination for computer workers

- visual training procedures that are useful for conditioning the eyes for the demands of VDT use
- stretching exercises for general relaxation

Chapter 6 summarizes the book and suggests possible long term solutions to the VDT visual stress problem.

KEY POINTS

* Our eyes are adapted for distance viewing, but modern cultural and economic demands are placing increased emphasis on close-up viewing.
* Our society is becoming increasingly dependent on computers and more people are spending time viewing video display terminals.
* Concerns over VDT-related health effects are increasing and many computer users report eye problems.
* Additional research is needed on VDT-related health effects. Scientific study will provide information needed for establishing guidelines for VDT use.

CHAPTER 2 - COMPUTER-EYE INTERACTION

Although the computer is a technological marvel, few devices since the Puritan "stocks" can compare with it for keeping man tethered to his work environment. As the Information Age requires that more and more of the population spend extended periods focusing on VDT's, there has been a corresponding increase in computer-related complaints. Before delving into the visual stress symptoms resulting from computer use, let's describe the functioning of a typical computer.

COMPUTER SYSTEM

The computer system that most people are familiar with consists of a computer, video display terminal, and keyboard. In the case of personal computers, the computer, VDT, and keyboard are all located on the same desk. Larger computer systems may have a central computer located in a remote location with multiple terminals networked to it from various office locations. There may be a variety of other peripheral devices connected to the system, such as printers or disk drives, but for simplicity sake we will consider this abbreviated system (see Figure 1).

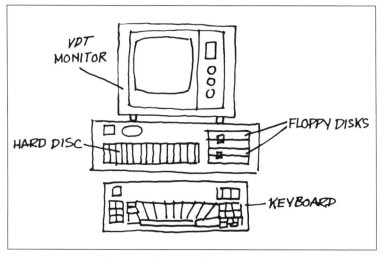

Figure 1. Typical Computer System

The "brains" of the system are located in the microprocessor chips(s) found within the computer itself. The microprocessor performs the information processing. The user must be able to communicate with the computer to tell it what to do. The most common input device is a keyboard, but others such as a **mouse, digitizer,** or **speech recognition** subsystem may be used. The VDT displays information input and/or output by the computer system

Sight, sound, and touch play varying roles in the human-computer interface. Touch is important for striking input keys or moving a mouse input device. Sound can enhance computer programs by adding speech, sound effects, or music. User input behavior can be regulated by warning or reinforcing sounds. For instance, a "beep" at an incorrect keyboard entry can alert the user about the error. In the future as speech recognition systems mature, sound may become a more important sense for interacting with computers. However, sight is the primary sense used to process the information generated by the computer system. We depend on our eyes to interpret the visual images displayed on the VDT.

A computer monitor, or VDT, is nothing more than a simple television screen. Inside is a **cathode ray tube (CRT)** which shoots a stream of electrons towards the back of the display screen surface (see Figure 2). The video display screen has a phosphor coating which emits light when struck by the electron beam. The light patterns cause text and graphic images to appear on the screen.

On a normal video screen, text displays as light characters against a dark background **(normal polarity)**. The phosphor coating is constantly refreshed by the electron

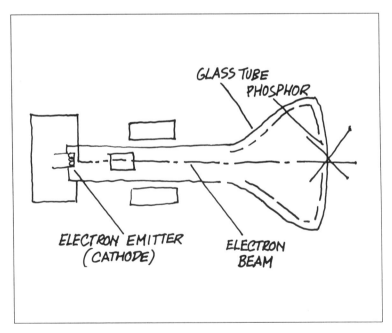

Figure 2. Cathode-Ray Tube

beam to prevent the screen image from fading. To maintain good display sharpness and avoid character "flicker" on the screen, the screen must be refreshed at least 60 times per second (60 Hertz). This is accomplished by a "sweeping" action of the electron beam across and down the screen at the refresh rate. For "reverse polarity" screen display (dark characters on a light background; analogous to printed page) a refresh rate of 80 Hertz is needed because flicker is more apparent on the larger light background area.

ANATOMY & PHYSIOLOGY OF THE EYE

While discussing computer technology, it is helpful to go into a little detail on the anatomy of the eye and its functioning during computer use. The eyes are our gateway to the world around us. The eyes gather visual images and pass them to the brain which synthesizes the information into a picture of the physical environment around us at any given instant. Vision also provides the foundation for our intellectual development through reading and writing.

Light enters the eye through an adjustable aperture known as the **iris** (see Figure 3). The iris is the pigmented portion of the eye and determines eye color (blue, brown, hazel, etc.). In the center of the iris is a black opening, the **pupil,** which is made larger or smaller by muscles that control the amount of light entering the eye. You can test the responsiveness of your eyes to light levels by standing in front of your bathroom mirror and observing the size of your pupils while switching the lights on and off.

The lens focuses light entering the eye onto the photo-receptive area (**retina**) in the rear of the eye. The lens can either elongate or shorten to provide the proper adjust-

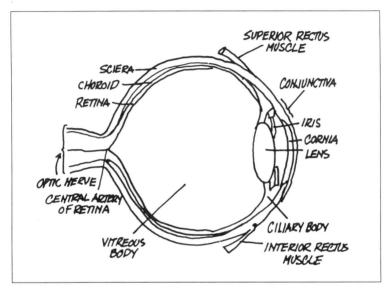

Figure 3. Cross-section of the Eye

ment needed to clearly focus an image on the retina. The retina has photo-receptor cells (primarily **rods** and **cones**) which may be thought of as an extension of our brain. These cells are sensitive to light and record the visual images that the eye sees. The rods function primarily for low light conditions and are responsible for differentiating between shades of grey and black. The cones function in higher illumination situations, such as normal daylight, and their primary role is to differentiate between colors. Together, the rods and cones process light images and create a neurological "picture" for the mind to interpret.

There are a series of six muscles controlling the external movement of the eye. Figure 4 shows these muscles and Table 2 lists their functions. Muscles often act in opposition, for example the **biceps** muscle flexes the arm, while the **triceps** muscles straightens the arm. Such is the case with the eye muscles. The **obliquus inferior** and the **rectus superior** act together to rotate the eyeball directly upward; the **obliquus superior** and the **rectus inferior** turn it directly downward. The **rectus lateralis** turns the eyeball directly outward, and the **rectus medialis** turns the eyeball inward.

Let's consider some of the ways VDT use can lead to eye strain and eye muscle fatigue. Throughout the day eye muscles are constantly positioning the eye. As we read a line of text the eyes must track from left to right and then back again. Scanning the computer display screen calls for up and down eye movement as well.

As we sit at the computer and shift our attention from screen to the printed copy or to look around the office, we must refocus our eyes. Each time we change our focusing distance the **ciliary** muscles must modify the shape of the lens to insure that a clear image appears on the retina. Shifting from a dimly lit display screen to the brightly background of the office requires changing the pupil size. In the iris, **radial** muscles dilate and **circular** muscles constrict the pupil size.

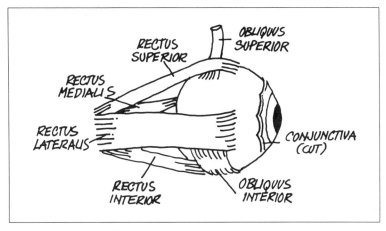

Figure 4. Eye Movement Muscles

MUSCLE NAME	EYE MOVEMENT FUNCTION
Rectus medialis	Inward
Rectus lateralis	Outward
Obliquus superior	Outward and downward
Rectus inferior	Inward and downward
Obliquus inferior	Outward and upward
Rectus superior	Inward and upward

Table 2. Eye Movement Muscles and Function

Eye fatigue also stems from the static muscle load required to keep the eyes focused on the screen with little movement for extended periods. Imagine holding your arm out from your body. Alright for a minute or two, but a longer time causes the arm to feel like its made of lead. A computer programmer, concentrating on the display screen while trying to find the "bug" in a line of code, may experience a similar discomfort, resulting from static eye muscle overload.

Left - right - up - down - near - far - bright - dim --- its easy to see how our eyes get the type of daily workout that clearly would make any aerobics instructor happy. Unfortunately because of the visually demanding nature of VDT use, these muscles are too often getting pushed to overload. Moderate exercise is fine; too much is harmful. Fatigue sets in, our ability to concentrate diminishes, the pressure of a job deadline lingers, and the result can be eyestrain, headaches, irritability, lowered productivity, and a stressful work environment that can carry over to the home and outside activities.

Models of Vision

Optometrists have proposed various models of vision to explain how the eye processes visual images. The most common models used to describe vision are the traditional, medical, and behavioral. These models have different advocates and describe the visual process in a different manner.

The **traditional** (sometimes called classical) **model** of vision contends that the ability of a person to see clearly at distance is a measure of good vision. Our ancestors depended on excellent distance vision for hunting food and avoiding predators. However, in the modern world distance viewing is less important. In the last fifty years, the US economy has shifted from industrial to knowledge intensive. As man has become more literate, the ability to use the eyes at near distances is increasingly a necessity.

The **medical model** of vision attempts to correlate visual problems with diseases, genetics, and physical conditions that affect eyesight. The "healthy" eye should be able to process visual information either close-up or at distance without any evidence of pathological problems. Based on the medical model, judging adverse effects of VDT use involves looking for evidence of eye diseases, hereditary factors or physical problems. This model also falls short in explaining the many complaints found in healthy, disease free users.

The **behavioral model**, developed in the last fifty years, is the most recent and complete model used to explain vision. The behavioral model has its foundation in a branch of optometry, known as **behavioral optometry**. Behavioral optometrists believe that vision is a learned and complex developmental process. As such, our environment and interactions with other senses can influence our vision. The behavioral model of vision derives from a wide variety of fields, including optometry, nutrition, child development, psychology, neurology, and physiology.

KEY POINTS

* The VDT uses a cathode ray tube to create a screen display. This is the same technology used in most TV sets.
* Users interact with the computer primarily using vision.
* Computer-eye interaction places heavy demands on our visual system.

CHAPTER 3 - VISUAL STRESS SYMPTOMS

Productivity gains through computer use are clearly not without a price. The increasing number of health-related complaints attributed to computer use give testimony to the detrimental side effects of prolonged computer use. However since computers are such valuable tools, it is unlikely that their usage will decline. Instead, we must devise ways with which to cope with the drawbacks of this new technology.

/Visual discomfort is the most common problem reported by VDT workers and this can be a key factor in reducing job productivity. Visual skills such as eye movement, focusing, and binocular vision (both eyes working in tandem) are essential for the intellectual development of most individuals. Visual stress can affect concentration and the ability to understand work or educational material, because of the emphasis humans place on vision for learning./

At present there are several ways in which workers can deal with computer-induced visual stress (Figure 5). One way to cope is to avoid doing any work requiring close-up sight at all. In another case, workers may perform the work, but with reduced comprehension while experiencing physical discomfort. Finally, workers may function in a visually stressful environment by developing maladaptations to the stress. This could include nearsightedness or the shutting off of vision from one eye (suppression of vision).

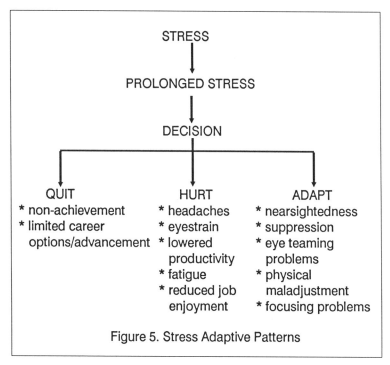

Figure 5. Stress Adaptive Patterns

Obviously none of these adaptive patterns are productive and some may be harmful to the long term health of the individual. People must become more aware of the consequences of extended VDT use and learn ways of dealing with the stress associated with computer usage.

Direct signs of visual stress include symptoms such as eyestrain, headaches, focusing difficulty, nearsightedness, doubling of vision, and changes in color perception. Indirect symptoms of visual stress may include musculo-skeletal pains (neck, shoulder, back, wrist), excessive physical fatigue, and lowered visual efficiency and job performance.

Eye Strain and Related Visual Problems

There has been much debate lately about whether or not VDT operation is harmful to one's eyes. According to a report by a panel of experts assembled by the National Research Council, there is no permanent damage to one's eyes while working with a VDT.[7] In the 1983 report, Panel Chairman Edward Rinalducci states "Our general conclusion is that eye discomfort, blurred vision and other visual disturbances, muscular aches, and stress reported among VDT workers are probably not due to anything inherent in VDT technology. It seems likely that with proper design of VDT display characteristics, workplace lighting, work stations and jobs, VDT work need not cause any unique visual problems." Another Panel member, neurologist Lawrence Stark states, "All the complaints of burning, eyestrain, headache, stinging, watery eyes connected with VDT use are valid claims. Just because you cannot measure visual fatigue does not mean it does not exist." This quote by Stark points out that even among Panel members the report's conclusions met with some dissent. A general area of agreement among the panel members highlights the need for more controlled (properly designed) studies. These studies will help determine if there is a causal link between computer use and eye problems.

There exists another group of professionals, **behavioral optometrists,** that contend that the 1983 National Research Council Committee on Vision claims are invalid.

Many behavioral optometrists feel they can clinically measure visual fatigue. They believe many **refractive errors** (the need for corrective lenses) are a consequence of near point visual stress. **Visual stress** is an internal dissonance that an individual attempts to resolve in some manner (i.e., avoidance, discomfort, maladaptation). A major cause of visual stress is a breakdown between the coordination of the focusing and eye alignment systems.

Visual stress results in the inability of a person to process light information in a comfortable, efficient manner. For the majority of individuals operating a VDT, visual stress has become a very real issue affecting working behaviors. VDT use places a great demand on **accommodation** (eye focusing), **ocular motility** (eye movement skills), **convergence** (bringing the eyes together at close range), and **binocularity** (using both eyes as a team). Clinical optometry has proven that these visual skills are dynamic and can breakdown depending upon excessive use and environmental stresses. Models of vision within behavioral optometry also indicate that the visual skills VDT workers use are learned and developed visual abilities. These visual abilities can be improved through appropriate visual training.

Many individuals who use computers for long periods continuously (more than 2 hours per day) complain of visual problems. Evidence suggests that the VDT is the primary cause of these eye problems. Table 3 taken from a study of VDT health complaints gives a comparison of VDT versus non-VDT usage visual stress symptoms.[8] The information in Table 3 indicates that VDT users complain of a greater number of visual stress problems.

VDT vs NON-VDT USAGE VISION COMPLAINTS

Complaint	Percentage of clerical workers **using** VDTs who expressed this complaint	Percentage of clerical workers **not using** VDTs who expressed this complaint
CHANGES IN COLOR PERCEPTION	40	9
IRRITATED EYES	74	47
BURNING EYES	80	44
BLURRED VISION	71	35
EYESTRAIN	91	60

Table 3. Comparison of VDT vs non-VDT usage vision complaints (from Smith et al. 1981)

Other studies have linked vision problems to VDT usage. Daily VDT users may develop chronic vision problems. A study of clerical workers (Table 4) showed a positive correlation between the number of hours a day spent using a VDT and the number of stress symptoms.[9] There is also evidence that an increase in the number of stress symptoms occurs based on the time duration workers spent on a VDT without a break.

Table 4. Hours of VDT Usage and Reported Health Problems
=============================

Health	Hours of VDT Usage Per Week		
	< 15 HRS.	15-30 HRS.	> 30 HRS.
Eyestrain *	33%	37%	63%
Headache	20%	27%	47%
Nausea	4%	6%	5%
Trouble Sleeping	13%	11%	11%
Back Pain	23%	26%	40%
Neck Pain	18%	23%	33%
Arm Pain	13%	19%	19%
Shoulder Pain	23%	20%	26%
Fatigue *	28%	28%	52%
Stomach Pain	10%	12%	14%
Skin Rashes	5%	1%	0%
Rapid Breathing	5%	3%	2%
Chest Pain	10%	9%	9%
Tension	21%	16%	11%
Anger	1%	4%	5%
Depression	6%	2%	5%
Menstrual Problems	3%	5%	7%
Vision Problems	3%	5%	12%

=============================
* $p < 0.05$ (from Resko & Mansfield, 1987)

Eye Focusing Problems

For optimal viewing comfort the VDT screen should display information at a distance upon which the human eye can focus comfortably for longer periods. Research into how computer use affects the eyes' ability to focus has uncovered a phenomena known as "**lag**" (see Figure 6). Although, not a new concept to optometry, lag has taken on new significance in its influence on VDT users. A simplistic definition for lag is that it represents the "difference between the distance of the material being viewed and the distance at which the viewer naturally focuses."[10]

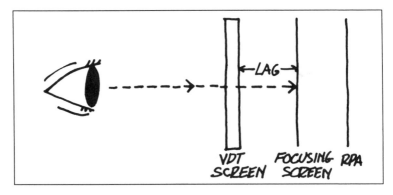

Figure 6. Lag & Resting Point of Accommodation

Another related concept is the "**resting point of accommodation.**" The resting point of accommodation (RPA) "is the point at which a person focuses their eyes when they are looking into a featureless visual field."[11] Theoretical optometry contends that the resting point of accommodation occurs when the eye focuses on infinity (at the horizon). More recent information suggests that individuals have a characteristic resting point of accommodation that varies within individuals and is less than infinity.[12]

The RPA acts as an index of visual fatigue. In suboptimal viewing conditions the eye focus tends to shift away from the ideal focal length required to view an object and move towards the RPA. As this occurs, the visual images on the screen become more difficult to see.

An ergonomic researcher, Gerald Murch, used laser technology to investigate visual fatigue in computer users over time.[13] The laser measured the focal length of eyes viewing a display screen. Comparing the clinically determined eye focal length with the actual distance of the viewed object determines the amount of visual lag. Murch's findings indicate that the eye cannot focus on the information displayed on a VDT screen with the same accuracy as the printed page. Instead when viewing a VDT over a period of hours the eye's focusing point extends beyond the display screen and approaches the RPA. This increase in visual lag over time when viewing the VDT results in a degradation of the screen image. The viewer must then expend extra effort to both focus on and process visual information. The results indicate that the images on the VDT screen do not provide enough stimulus to allow for optimal eye accommodation. The results of an RPA measurement can indicate the need for corrective action. Specially prescribed VDT glasses and/or visual training allow sharp focus of the VDT screen.

The need to change focus between the screen, printed copy, and office environment intensifies the problem. This behavior places heavy demands on the focusing abilities of the eye and its associated muscles.

Clinical optometrists have also reported that certain individuals respond in a different manner to a VDT screen by overfocusing; as if the screen distance was much closer to them than the actual physical distance. This type of persistent overfocusing (clinically referred to as accommodative spasms) can result in degradation in screen images leading to maladaptations in visual function. This often results in lowered speed and comprehension while working with VDTs.

Nearsightedness

Nearsightedness, or **myopia**, is a common visual problem in our society. Typically, nearsighted individuals see clearly at a close range, but experience blurred vision when viewing at far distances. Approximately 36% of Americans require prescription lenses to neutralize myopia and attain normal distance clarity, or so called 20/20 vision.

Today debate revolves around whether the genetic makeup of an individual causes myopia, or whether myopia develops because of environmental stresses affecting the eyes. Poor visual environmental conditions (such as improper lighting, poor posture, reading at distances close enough to cause undo stress) are possible factors contributing to myopia.

Behavioral optometrists strongly favor the argument that most myopia develops because of the need to adapt to close range visual stresses. Research suggests that the human visual system initially developed for distant viewing abilities. Only in the last 200 years or so have humans needed to use their eyes for a preponderance of close tasks; particularly in this age of computer generated information. Evolutionary changes of the visual system have yet to compensate for all of these close working demands. So, as an adaptation to close range vision difficulties, a nearsighted condition develops to reduce the demands of looking at close ranges.

Perhaps the only advantage of myopia is a comfortable ability to function at close reading ranges. The disadvantages, such as blurred distance vision, increased incidence of certain eye diseases (most notably retinal detachment), and the need to wear prescription glasses for driving, flying, etc., clearly outweigh the one advantage. To avoid the development of myopia we must pay attention to appropriate visual hygiene while reading, studying, or viewing computer displays. Visual hygiene is discussed in Chapter 5.

Changes in Color Perception

Some VDT users have reported a change in color perception after extended computer use. Viewing the display screen constantly for long periods, and then shifting the eyes to a lighter viewing background may result in an "afterglow." The user may perceive colors that are opposite or complementary to those of the display screen background. For example, steadily viewing a green screen monitor may lead to a pink color perception when shifting focus. Although this phenomenon can be alarming, it is harmless and disappears after a short time.

Doubling of Vision

Some VDT users have reported a doubling of images after working long periods with a computer. **Diplopia** (or double vision) is due to the breakdown of eye coordination skills. The condition is usually temporary, and normal vision will return by resting the eyes. Sudden and persistent episodes of double vision should be immediately evaluated by an eyecare professional to rule out serious neurological dysfunction.

"Dry Eye" Syndrome

Many computer users wear contact lenses and are susceptible to a condition known as "dry eye" syndrome. The tendency to concentrate on the computer screen suppresses the normal eye blinking reflex. This can contribute to deposit build up and to drying of the lenses. The low humidity environment that computer workstations require and static attraction of dust to the screen area can exacerbate this situation. To correct this dry eye problem, optometrists suggest frequent eye lubrication while wearing contact lenses. The VDT user should consult an eyecare professional if dry eye symptoms persist.

Vision and Posture

Numerous posture-related problems relate to visual stress. If an individual is lacking in the visual skills needed to align, track, and focus on an image, then the body may compensate by substituting head for eye movements. The suboptimal viewing conditions that many times accompany VDT use intensify problems in this area. Head, neck, shoulder, hand, and back pain complaints are common among many workers using VDT terminals (see Figure 7).[14, 15]

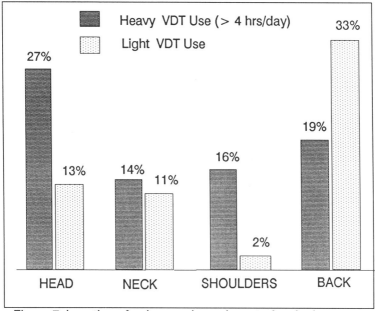

Figure 7. Location of pain experienced most often by heavy and light VDT use groups (from Fahrbach and Chapman, 1990).

VDTs and Stress

The amount of stress we experience at work depends on our job type and individual nature. Some job types are inherently more stressful than others. More difficult to measure is the individual's response to stress. Some people cope quite well in stressful situations, while others may get "stressed-out" at the slightest provocation. Regardless of these variables, it is certain that all workers experience some degree of on the job stress.

/ Stress can affect vision. Visual stress reactions can be observed by measuring alpha brain wave patterns. In visually stressful environments the alpha waves show increased amplitude. This is similar to increased background noise, like record scratches, that may detract from the music appreciation of a stereo listener. The "visual noise" shown in these brain wave patterns is not conducive for understanding visual information.

Dr. J.R. Pierce of the University of Alabama observed physiological evidence of visual stress.[16] Like other stresses, visual stress produced changes in heartbeat, respiration, galvanic skin response, along with other physiological stress indicators. These physiological changes demonstrate an immediate response to environmental stresses.

A person under stress is apt to find that his or her ability to concentrate on a work task is impaired. This can lead to increased errors and lowered productivity. Excessive chronic exposure to stress can result in more severe mental or social problems, including anxiety, depression, fatigue, irritability, moodiness, general job "burn-out", low productivity, and high absenteeism.[17,18].

Studies of VDT operators suggest a relationship between job type and stress levels.[19] Often, the job design, and not the worker, is the cause of stress. VDT users such as air traffic controllers and data entry clerks are at the high end of the visual stress spectrum (see Figure 8). Jobs like these are often closely timed and monitored, repetitive, and socially isolated, all characteristics which contribute to a high stress level. Jobs that provide more latitude for the worker to control job pacing and design of the work are the easiest to deal with. For this reason, it is not surprising that most professionals and executives report the least amount of stress associated with VDT use.

VISUAL STRESS	JOB
HIGH	Air Traffic Control Data Entry Accountant Word Processor
MEDIUM	Secretary (fulltime) Secretary (parttime) Editor Author
LOW	Executive

Figure 8. Visual Stress Spectrum for VDT-Related Jobs
(Reprinted with permission OEP Foundation, Santa Ana, CA)

Table 5 presents information on the relationship between VDT job tasks and factors including keyboard input rate, visual emphasis, job pacing, and decision making. The table shows that jobs vary considerably in terms of computer interaction. Data entry tasks require a high keyboard input rate, usually according to a fixed input format. The visual emphasis is on the source document, with the VDT operator checking the screen periodically to verify input. Data acquisition include jobs like telephone information operators. These jobs involve computer information retrieval with the visual emphasis on the screen only. Interactive communication tasks combines both data entry and acquisition work. Airline reservation personnel fall into this task category. Word processing encompasses many of the tasks involved in secretarial work, including document formatting and text entry, correction, search, and recall.

Table 5. Some Video Display Terminal Task Categories

TASK CATEGORY	INPUT RATE (Strokes/Min)	VISUAL EMPHASIS	INTERRUPTIONS	WORK SPEED CONTROL	DECISION MAKING
Data entry	High	Source document (screen/copy/screen checks)	Very few	Little to none	Little
Data acquisition	Medium	Screen only	Some	Varies	Some
Interactive Communication	Medium/ intermittent	Screen only (some keyboard)	Lags for processing	Varies	Some
Word processing	High/ intermittent	Screen/copy	Few	Some	Varies
Programming	Low/ intermittent	Copy/screen	Frequent	Much	Great
CAD/CAM	Low/ intermittent	Screen/copy	Frequent	Much	Great

Video Displays, Works, and Vision, copyright 1983, by the National Academy of Sciences, National Academy Press, Washington, DC.

Many jobs (writers, editors, proofreaders) include word processing tasks. Programming and CAD/CAM (computer-assisted design/computer-assisted manufacturing) job tasks involve varying amounts of daily computer use. These workers have considerable job control and authority to make decisions. Many scientific and professional jobs fit this profile.

In addition to the work organization, other environmental and physical conditions in the workplace can have a contributing and compounding effect on the degree of stress experienced. Factors leading to job stress include poor lighting, excessive noise levels, unhealthy air quality, inadequate work space, and poorly designed furniture and workstations.

KEY POINTS

* Computer-induced visual stress is a common
   workplace problem
* There are a variety of direct and indirect symptoms
   associated with computer-induced visual stress.
   Symptoms include eyestrain, eye focusing difficulties,
   nearsightedness, changes in color perception, double
   vision, musculo-skeletal pains, and general stress.
* Lack of awareness about visual stress reducing
   methods often causes VDT users to deal with the
   problem in an unproductive or unhealthy manner.
   Adverse response patterns to VDT-induced visual
   stress include job avoidance, discomfort, or vision
   maladaptations.

CHAPTER 4 - THE VDT WORKING ENVIRONMENT AND VISUAL STRESS

The number of vision complaints reported relates to the computer working environment. A report by the National Academy of Science suggested that an improvement of ergonomic condition alone could reduce worker complaints by up to 39 percent (see Figure 9).[20]

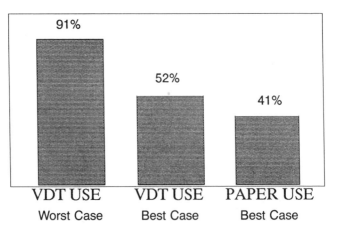

Figure 9. Comparison of vision-related complaints reported by VDT operators in different work environments (from VDTs and Vision, OEP Report, 1985)

In general, workers viewing a VDT screen reported more vision complaints compared with those viewing printed material (paper use).

Often the computer is unpacked from its box, placed on a flat surface, and plugged in, without any regard for ergonomic considerations. There may be all sorts of harmful effects - glare, reflections, poor lighting, etc. It's no wonder vision problems result. Setting up the computer workstation in the proper manner can reduce or eliminate visual stress.

The computer work environment encompasses a diverse group of factors, including lighting, user position, computer placement, noise, and air quality. Although it is difficult to quantify some of these factors, they all contribute to the stress level of using the computer.

Aside from the physical characteristics of the work environment, there are additional aspects of a job that can contribute to visual stress. These include job design and organization, the physiological and psychological profile of the VDT user, the visual efficiency of the operator, and the characteristics of the VDT workstation.

One of the goals of behavioral optometry is to reduce or eliminate environmental parameters that may lead to visual stress. Studies have estimated that only 5 - 10% of all VDT users work under fully satisfactory ergonomic conditions.[21] There is evidence that a variety of changes in the workplace can improve the visual comfort of VDT operators. Let's consider some of the factors of the overall VDT working environment that can have a detrimental effect on the computer user.

COMPUTER SYSTEM

VDT Screen Display Characteristics

Flat Two-Dimensional Displays. The computer requires a fundamental change in our orientation to text processing. The computer substitutes illuminated characters on the computer screen for the printed page. In addition, we focus down when reading a printed page. The traditional work environment requires lowering the individual's line of sight 20-40 degrees to focus on the printed page or typewriter key. Rather than looking down we must shift our focus horizontally to view the VDT. This horizontal line of sight makes the viewer susceptible to more visual interference (e.g., glare, distracting background, variations in room light intensity). The screen may also act as a mirror reflecting nearby objects which further interferes with our vision (see later discussion on glare).

The natural position of our eyes at rest is a 20 degree downward gaze. The horizontal shift required to view a VDT screen increases muscle tonus around our eyes, which causes visual stress. In addition, the VDT often requires that we stare for extended periods at a flat two dimensional display. This provides little visual relief and may not provide enough eye stimulation to maintain proper focus.

Contrast Limitations. When computers first arrived on the scene many people felt left in the dark when dealing with this new technology. It turns out that being left in the dark is not so bad when viewing a computer screen.

The ability to read characters on a computer terminal is dependent on the contrast between the illuminated screen text and the screen background. A dimly illuminated work environment is best. With a dim background the eye has less adjusting to do. The computer screen has a low light intensity. When looking away from the screen the eyes must adjust to the varying degrees of brightness in the room. The usual office environment, brightly lit, forces the eye pupils to constrict to reduce the light input. Continually shifting between a darkened VDT screen and brightly lit background puts strain on the eye muscles and leads to fatigue. Darkening the work area allows the pupils to relax when looking away from the screen. This is a lot less stressful.

However, while a darkened work area may be conducive to viewing the VDT it creates problems when trying to read printed copy simultaneously. The solution is to use a desk lamp. This will relieve the starkness of a dimly lit room and provide illumination for reading. Keep in mind that the position of the desk lamp may be crucial to success. You must provide adequate print illumination, but avoid adding glare to the computer system.

Colors. Character appearance on the VDT screen can have a decided effect on the user's visual comfort. Red and blue screen characters are difficult to see and best avoided. The ideal colors for screen characters are in the middle of the light spectrum: green, yellow, and orange. Various other combinations are possible. Within these guidelines the VDT user should choose a screen color combination that is comfortable to view.

Polarity. Normally, the VDT screen displays light characters on a dark background. This polarity is familiar to most users and is similar to a film negative. Reverse polarity or reverse video (where dark characters appear on a light screen background) is another option and may be desirable for some. Reverse polarity corresponds to a printed page.

Research is inconclusive about whether normal video or reverse video is preferable. The user may try alternating between normal and reverse screen polarity during the day to provide eye stimulus variety.

Luminance. The computer terminal should allow adjustment of the screen character brightness. Ideally the characters should conform to the 10-3-1 standard contrast ratio. Experts suggest that characters on the screen should be 10 times brighter than the screen background and the ambient room lighting should be 3 times brighter than the screen background.[22] Using a camera light meter can help you obtain a fairly accurate contrast ratio at your workstation.

The operator should adjust screen brightness and contrast for maximum viewing comfort. Some VDT users have reported that varying the screen brightness during the day provides relief from eye fatigue.

Character Size and Type. Optimal character display size should provide for easy character resolution and the optimal display of information on the screen. A character height of between 2.5 mm and 3.0 mm is recommended and individual characters should be sharply defined on the screen. Industry standards call for 80 character lines with 25 lines per screen.

The resolution of screen characters are dependent on the **dot matrix** dimensions. Each element in the matrix is called a **pixel,** which stands for picture element (see Figure 10). The CRT's electron beam sweeps across the display screen and selectively excites pixels (phosphorus dots) to create screen characters. Matrix dimensions of 5 X 7, 7 X 9, and 9 X 11 are common. The higher the dot matrix, the better the character quality. Characters composed of a dot matrix of at least 7 X 9 are best.

Font type has a bearing on the legibility of screen text. Some font types are inherently more difficult to decipher on the VDT screen. The VDT cathode ray tube corresponds to the technology used on the TV screen. Just like on a TV, small, poorly defined text is difficult to see on a VDT screen.

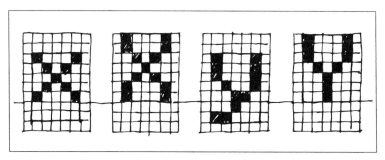

Figure 10. Screen Characters Displayed in a 5 X 7 Dot Matrix

Check the VDT every six months to make certain the device is operating within the manufacturer's specifications. Refer to the manufacturer's recommended maintenance suggestions for information on how to conduct periodic inspections. The inspection will also insure proper text character quality.

Scrolling. New information may scroll onto the screen line by line from the screen bottom or may appear a page at a time. Information should display at a rate which is conducive to comprehension. The viewer must be aware of how information appears, and adjust tracking and scanning visual skills accordingly. This skill can vary dramatically among operators.

"Flicker" and "Swim." Screen "flicker" and "swim" are problems caused by VDT malfunctioning. Characters on the screen may flicker, distracting the operator's concentration. One factor contributing to flicker is the screen character "refresh" rate (the number of times per second the screen phosphor repaints). If the refresh rate is less than 60 Hertz for normal polarity display or 80 Hertz for reverse polarity display, then character flicker may become noticeable.

"Swim" refers to the movement of the screen display in its entirety in a wave-like fashion, usually in a vertical direction. Maintenance service can correct VDT swim problems.

Screen characters may appear blurred, especially when compared with printed copy. Poor character quality combined with screen flicker or swim forces the eyes to constantly adjust to varying light levels. This tires the eye muscles and leads to visual fatigue. If the viewer is very sensitive to these problems, then the only solution may be to replace the guilty terminal. Fortunately, recent advances in technology has virtually eliminated flicker and swim in computer systems made since 1989.

Screen Filter. Filters are available that cover the VDT screen and help eliminate the glare, static, and radiation problems associated with VDT viewing.

Glare caused from lighting fixtures, windows, or reflections can "wash out" characters on portions of the VDT screen. Glare makes the eyes work harder, adjusting to the varying light intensities, and this leads to eye fatigue. Filters cut down on glare in several ways. Some screens have anti-reflective coatings that can absorb light before it strikes the screen. Filters with polarizing properties trap light reflected from the screen and help enhance character contrast. There are mesh screens that act like a louver preventing incoming light from hitting the screen, while allowing light emitted from the VDT to travel unimpeded for glare-free viewing. Be aware that some filters make the screen darker and reduce character readability, causing a tradeoff between improved screen visibility and diminished character resolution.

The electromagnetic property of VDT screens leads to static build-up. Discharge from static shocks can destroy data and damage computer equipment. Static also causes dust and smoke particles to collect on the screen and this leads to poor vision. To remedy this situation, some filters have a permanent, conductive coating to dissipate static buildup. Grounding cords help drain away static charges and electromagnetic radiation. Screens without anti-static features should be cleaned daily using an anti-static spray or cloth. Anti-static dust covers are also useful for dissipating static charge and preventing dust collection when the computer is not in use.

Computer terminals emit electromagnetic radiation at low levels (soft X-ray, very low and extremely low frequency radiation) that can be a cause of health concern. Some filters have radiation absorbing properties. However, because radiation emanates from all surfaces of the terminal and travels in circular patterns, it is nearly impossible to stop with a simple filter.

The best filters provide high contrast and resolution, and have anti-glare, anti-static, and anti-radiation properties. Filters range in price from about $20 to near $200, and their price reflects the amount of protection they provide. Computer monitors that emit no radiation are also available. A VDT visor is an economical means of controlling glare problems. The visor fits over the terminal top and reduces glare and reflections.

VDT Keyboard

Keyboard attributes can cause discomfort while using the computer. Factors, such as keyboard layout, key size, keyboard angle and height, key press resistance, and colors used to separate key functions, can enhance or deter VDT usability. Poorly designed keyboards are linked to Repetitive Strain Injury, a problem that causes wrist pain. A detachable keyboard which allows its comfortable positioning in relation to the computer is desirable. Avoid terminals that have directly attached keyboards because they provide little latitude to accommodate comfortable viewer positioning.

Working Distance

The VDT viewing distance (18 - 25 inches) is greater than the normal reading distance (12 - 16 inches). This forces an increase in the normal eye focal length used for reading. Take a book and start reading it at a distance that feels comfortable. Now, move the book out to about twice the distance. That gives you some idea of the focal length used in viewing the VDT.

The average of all viewing distance recommendations is 20 inches (50 cm).[23] The line of sight to the top of the screen is 20 degrees below horizontal and the line of sight to the bottom of the screen 20 degrees lower (see Figure 11).

Special "terminal viewing" glasses can aid users for proper focus on the computer screen. As time goes on, "terminal viewing" glasses may become a common tool for computer users. Computer eyeglasses are prescription glasses and are discussed in more detail in Chapter 5.

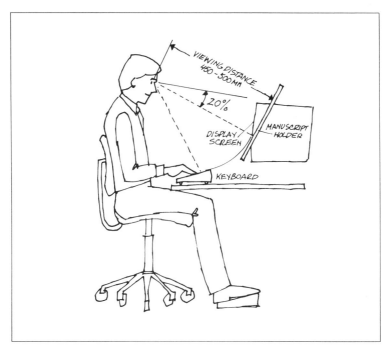

Figure 11. Recommended VDT Viewing Distance

Furniture and Work Space Design

The type and design of furniture used with the computer workstation can influence the visual and general comfort of the user. Avoid chairs that are uncomfortable and require awkward body positioning to view the VDT or access the keyboard. This can lead to aches and pains. Postural problems which result in wrist, neck, shoulder, or back problems are often indirect signs of visual stress.

The seat used with the VDT workstation should be adjustable. Pneumatically adjustable chairs with back support are excellent. Adjust the chair to support the lower back (lumbar). A swivel chair with a sturdy base on casters, is also a good choice.

The computer terminal should be on a tilt-and-swivel base for adjusting its position to eliminate glare and screen reflections. A copy holder that can be positioned at the same distance as the terminal screen is also helpful for comfortable viewing while entering text or data. The copy may also be placed under the display between the screen and keyboard.

There are numerous computer desk or workstation designs. The workstation should fit your needs and allow you to perform your job in a comfortable, efficient manner. The workstation or surrounding work space should provide adequate shelves and filing cabinets. There should be ready access to frequently used equipment, such as the printer or the telephone.

If you have some control over your work space design, consider how you can integrate privacy, comfort, and functionality to create an optimal work environment. You may want to consult computer supply catalogs or discuss your needs with computer furniture dealers to get an idea of the available options.

PHYSICAL CHARACTERISTICS OF THE WORK ENVIRONMENT

Glare

Glare - you've experienced it on a sunny day particularly if you ski or spend time at the beach. Glare is often more subtle when viewing a computer monitor, but can be an important source of visual stress.

Computers are often situated in work environments where overhead lights or uncurtained windows may be glare-producing sources. Although identifying sources of glare may be easy, their elimination is often more difficult. Putting curtains on a window is usually undesirable. Another approach is to either move the computer terminal away from the glare or to add partitions to remove the unwanted glare. Anti-glare screen filters are also useful for correcting this problem.

Room Temperature

Computers generate heat. In confined quarters a group of computers can make the room temperature uncomfortably warm. At the other extreme in an air-conditioned environment the sedentary nature of computer work can make it feel like frostbite is setting in. These factors can act as indirect stressors affecting the concentration and the visual performance of the VDT user.

Air Quality

The electrical characteristics of computers make it advisable to keep them in a low humidity environment. Low humidity can lead to "dry eye" syndrome in contact lens wearers. A smokey room can be a major source of eye irritation. Most work places today are "smoke-free" and the importance of this cannot be overemphasized. Other air quality conditions can be detrimental to worker performance. Stale or oppressively humid air affects the ability to carry out productive work for lengthy periods.

Room Illumination

Lighting in the room should be 3 times brighter than the screen background. Most office lighting is too bright for optimal VDT screen viewing. If possible, turn off overhead lights to darken the room environment and reduce light reflection. Use desk lighting instead of overhead for reading printed copy.

The optimal light intensity is about half of the 50 to 100 footcandles found in most "typing pool" rooms. The less contrast there is between the VDT screen and the surrounding background the better. This requires fewer eye focusing adjustments and reduces eye fatigue. If a light meter is available the recommended contrast ratio between the illuminated characters and screen background is 10:1.

Wall Surface and Color

Walls that are glossy can create distracting reflections that are annoying to the computer user. To create the best ambient room lighting conditions walls should have a flat "matte" finish preferably with a pastel color.

Visual Relief Area

VDT operators should face into an open space beyond the display screen. This provides an opportunity to focus occasionally on distant objects ("visual relief area") when looking away from the VDT.

If at all possible, avoid seating that has you looking into a windowless corner. In this case it is best to get up and walk around periodically to allow the eyes to focus on distant objects.

Noise

Unless you are next to a train station or construction site, there should be a noticeable reduction in noise level when switching from typewriter to computer usage. An exception may occur if you are in close proximity to a high impact printer (e.g., dot matrix printer). The printer should have a cover or box enclosure to reduce the noise level. Distractions from other workers may be a significant noise factor in some work environments. Noise can be an additional indirect factor that can intensify visual stress.

Reflected Images

The flat, two-dimensional VDT screen can act as a mirror reflecting objects or light sources in the surrounding area. Often the viewer may be unaware of annoying interference from screen reflections. Perform a "mirror test" to detect possible reflections. Face a mirror towards the VDT screen and move it slowly. Look to see if any bright images appear. If an interfering object is found, try to remove it or reduce its reflectance. If necessary, solve the problem by repositioning the screen or by applying a screen filter.

HUMAN OPERATOR

The physiological status of the VDT worker can influence the stress level experienced on the job. Good health is paramount for our enjoyment of all aspects of life. Individuals who enjoy a healthy existence will be able to perform well on the job and withstand the stress sometimes associated with VDT use. Because of the heavy demands VDT use can place on our visual system, it is important that the eyes be in good shape. Workers who have pre-existing eye problems, such as uncorrected refractive conditions, binocular vision problems or eye focusing problems, are likely to find them aggravated by VDT use.

Adult workers (over 40 years old) may experience a condition known as **presbyopia** where it is difficult to focus on near objects. This inevitable condition is a result of the decreased flexibility of the eye lens with age. A prescription for bifocals, trifocals, or reading glasses can compensate for this problem.

Perception of Work

The "pioneering spirit" associated with a new technology may have helped the initial computer users to cope with stresses accompanying VDT viewing. Since that time, the computer has pervaded almost every occupation in modern society and become a common tool. Accompanying increased computer usage is a seemingly exponential growth in VDT-related complaints. This is despite the fact that improvements are continually being made in workstation ergonomics.

Nowadays the initial glamour associated with computers has given way to a to a realization of the increased mechanization they bring to the workplace. This is particularly evident in environments where computers create a high demand and low control situation for the worker. The ability to monitor work output with computers can create undue stress in the individual worker. It is not surprising then that executives and white-collar professionals report the least VDT induced stress, while data entry and word processors experience the most.

The psychological profile of the worker can also influence job stress. How the worker perceives the job is an important factor determining stress levels. If a job environment meets a workers needs and abilities, then complaints are likely to be minimal. However, if there is a poor fit between the job and the worker's capability, then stress will result and is likely to be exaggerated by VDT use.

Contact Lenses

To avoid "dry eye" syndrome, contact lens wearers should consciously maintain normal blinking while using the VDT. The normal blinking rate is 6 - 15 times per minute. To help maintain eye moisture try to drink 6 - 8 glasses of water (or other liquids) a day. Additionally, it may be necessary to use lubricating eye drops to insure proper lens moisture. A cleaning during a mid-day break may also help to keep the lenses in optimal shape. Discuss these suggestions with your eyecare professional.

Terminal Spectacles (Computer Eyeglasses)

To accommodate the special demands that VDT viewing places on the user, optometrists can prescribe specialized eyeglasses. These eyeglasses, known as "terminal spectacles" or "computer eyeglasses," provide a better focus at typical screen distance (20 inches) and reduce visual stress.

A study of New York state employees conducted by the SUNY Center for Vision Care Policy found a significant improvement in eye comfort among workers wearing specially prescribed computer eyeglasses. After a year, nearly 94 percent of the workers noted an increase in eye comfort. In addition, 82 percent of the workers reported increased work efficiency.[24]

Routine eye exams may not be enough to alleviate the visual stress symptoms experienced by VDT users. Over 80 percent of the subjects in the New York study were already wearing corrective lenses.

It appears that computer eyeglasses may become occupational "tools" required for VDT users. Just as a welder is required to wear safety filter glasses, computer users may soon be donning terminal spectacles to perform their tasks. Traditionally prescribed and designed eyeglass lenses often do not provide adequate flexibility for computer viewing. Special computer bifocals have the top portion of the lens designed for screen viewing while the bottom portion is designed for viewing hard print copy. Trifocals are further specialized to provide lens areas for computer, text, and distance viewing. Discuss with your optometrist the pros and cons of various computer spectacle designs.

Eye Examinations and Visual Health

Computer operators should seek an evaluation of visual and ocular health on a yearly basis. The eye examination should be conducted by a licensed optometrist or ophthalmologist who is familiar with the visual demands of VDT use. Behavioral optometrists have specialized training which is useful for evaluating the visual needs of computer users.

"Behavioral optometrists spend years in post-graduate, continuing education to master the complex visual programs prescribed to prevent or eliminate visual problems and enhance visual performance.

Not all optometrists practice behavioral optometry, which includes developmental and functional optometry. If you do not now have an optometrist who practices behavioral optometry, call or write OEP Vision Extension (see Information Sources at end of the book). Or, make sure you receive a *yes* answer to each of the following questions before you make an appointment:

1. Do you make a full series of nearpoint vision tests?
2. Do you make work-related visual perception tests?
3. Do you provide full vision care and visual training in your office, or will you refer me to a colleague if needed?
4. Will you see me again during the year, and periodically to determine my progress?"

(Reprinted with permission, OEP Foundation, Santa Ana, CA)

Posture in Relation to the Workstation

The ideal situation should permit the following alignments simultaneously (see Figure 12):

1. Screen, copy, and console all at the same distance from the user's eyes. Copy holders are available to position a manuscript at the same distance as the computer screen.
2. Keep feet firmly on floor while seated. Short users may require a foot rest.
3. Trunk straight, but inclined forward about 20 degrees from the hips.
4. Keep wrists straight while typing on keyboard. Bending the wrist can lead to repetitive strain injury. Make sure wrists are not resting on sharp edge while typing.
5. Thighs horizontal with feet flat on the floor or on foot rest if necessary.

6. The upper arm should be vertical when using the VDT.
7. The forearm should be horizontal, or slightly lower, when operating the VDT.
8. The terminal and/or copy surfaces should be of such height that the upper surfaces of the thighs do not touch supporting undersurfaces.

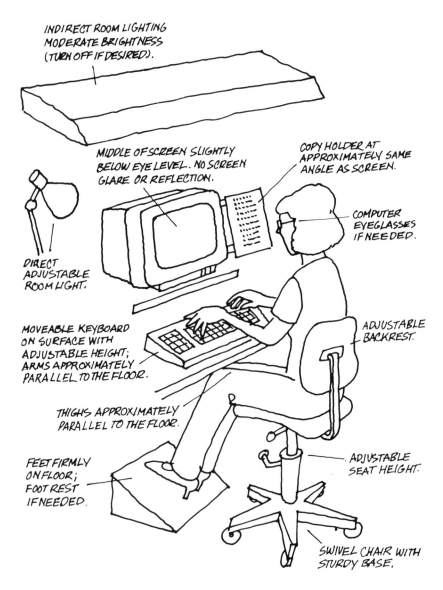

Figure 12. A Well Designed VDT Workstation

JOB DESIGN

Job design, in terms of structure, demands, and pace, can be another important influence on visual stress. There is a strong correlation between the visual demands of a job and worker reported visual discomfort. Factors, such as speed, complexity, vigilance, and workload, help determine the visual task demands of a job. Jobs that are complex or otherwise mentally demanding, require detailed vision and sustained concentration by the worker. This type of work can be visually and mentally fatiguing if carried on for too long a period without breaks or variation.

Jobs that are relatively straightforward, such as directory assistance or data entry, can also be stressful because of their structure and pace. This type of work is often repetitive and monotonous, which can prove tedious to an active mind. In addition, these jobs can be closely timed and monitored, often by computers. Management is able to quantify the performance of individual workers and this can lead to psychological as well as physical stress.

Varied Work

Studies show that workers who have little control over the content and speed of their work are susceptible to the greatest stress. Factors such a job duration, rest breaks, task variation, and job rotation influence the VDT user's stress level.

Other factors which can influence stress levels include the threat of job loss, predictability of events (computer breakdowns/delays) and social isolation.

Companies should make an effort to vary the tasks and pace of the daily job routine. This can dramatically improve employee productivity and health.

Rest Periods

A 15-minute break every two hours can improve vision and job productivity. Demanding VDT workloads usually require a short change (10-minute break) from VDT work each hour. Sometimes shorter, more frequent breaks (5 minutes or less) are helpful, especially if they can be taken at the worker's discretion.

During the break perform exercises at your desk or get up and take a walk. Visual training procedures and stretching exercises that are appropriate while at work are described in Chapter 5, Visual Training Techniques.

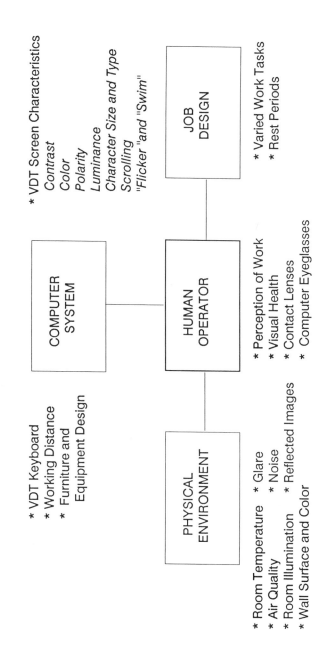

Figure 13. Summary Diagram of Factors in the VDT Working Environment Affecting Visual Stress

CHAPTER 5 - VISUAL TRAINING TECHNIQUES

There is a growing body of evidence that prolonged computer usage causes visual stress and creates undesirable visual adaptations. The sense of sight is a fragile system and crucial for maintaining intellectual development. Because of this, it is imperative that computer users become aware of proper visual hygiene while viewing video display screens. Before continuing our discussion of visual hygiene and introducing some of the visual training techniques useful for alleviating visual stress, let's summarize the basic philosophy underlying behavioral optometry.

This philosophy is based on the work of the late Dr. A.M. Skeffington, O.D., D.O.S., and his associates and promoted by the Optometric Extension Program Foundation (OEP). Founded in 1928, OEP is a nonprofit, post graduate education organization that fosters public awareness of the importance of vision and supports research in behavioral optometry. OEP summarizes behavioral optometry as follows:

"Behavioral optometry is a model of vision subscribed to by optometric practitioners around the world. According to the core concepts of that model, vision is a dynamic, dominant process directing the development of human behavior. As a dominant process, vision involves acquiring, monitoring, integrating, and modifying information and directing many action processes of the human. The human vision system is subject to adaptations and changes in function, and eventually changes in behavior, when subjected to persistent stresses. Many vision disorders are preventable. There are various regimens of care where optometrists can arrange conditions to allow individuals to operate at their highest level of performance. The primary methods used by behavioral optometry in preventative programs are nearpoint lenses, prisms, visual training programs and visual hygiene information."

(Reprinted with permission. OEP Foundation, Santa Ana, CA)

Visual training (vision therapy) is a method used to enable people to develop and enhance visual abilities. This can prevent vision problems. Vision problems and some eye problems are even reversible.

Optometrists have several avenues to pursue in treating vision disorders. Treatments include compensatory lenses (eyeglasses), prescription drugs, contact lenses, and vision therapy. The optometrist may apply these treatments individually, or in combinations, to achieve the desired state of eye health and visual efficiency.

All VDT users should have periodic eye examinations conducted by optometrists or ophthalmologists who are familiar with the visual demands of computer use. The examinations should occur at least on an annual basis. The examination provides an opportunity for the vision care professional to access how well your eyes are working for you. A proper eye examination for computer workers should address the following areas:

* ocular health,
* distance acuity
* near acuity
* how well eyes "team" (binocularity)
* how well you cope with near vision work
* assessment of focusing skills
* early signs or symptoms of visual stress

Eye examinations are important for diagnosing any eye diseases or related pathological problems. These types of health-related problems are relatively rare. The exam should also assess an individual's ability to see clearly at distance and close up. Finally, the examinations should evaluate a person's functional visual skills and their ability to do near vision work.

Specially prescribed computer eyeglasses have been shown to increase the comfort of VDT users. If your work involves extended periods of VDT use, you should discuss the need for computer eyeglasses with your vision care professional. Computer eyeglasses are for preventing eye problems and supplement any compensatory lenses you may now be using.

An example of specialized eyeglass lenses designed for computer users is shown in Figure 14. Trifocals are useful for certain individuals who have a need to focus on the VDT screen, read hard copy, and look in the distance during the course of their normal work. These occupational lens have three zones which accommodate the visual needs of the VDT user. Zone A is for distance viewing; zone B is for viewing the VDT; and zone C is for reading hard copy print. The division between lenses is fit relatively high to insure proper head positioning while viewing the

VDT. Bifocals are appropriate for jobs, such as word processors. The bifocal would consist of a reading lens (C) and an intermediate lens for viewing the VDT screen (B).

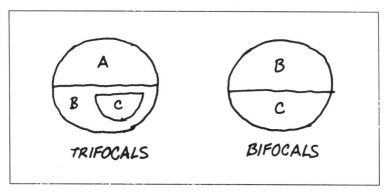

Figure 14. VDT Bifocals and Trifocals

The proper development of visual skills plays a key role in an individual's intellectual development. Using VDTs can place a heavy demand on the eyes. Therefore, it is crucial that visual skills are developed and functioning properly. The key visual skills for computer users are:

* Tracking   * Peripheral Vision
* Fixation   * Maintaining Attention
* Focus Change   * Near Vision Acuity
* Binocularity   * Visualization

For computer use, tracking, fixation, focus change, binocularity, maintaining attention, and near vision acuity skills are especially important. The VDT user must be able to scan text on the screen (tracking), fixate on individuals characters or words, and change focus rapidly back and forth between screen and printed copy (or near and far).

The eyes must be able to work in tandem (binocularity) for stress free viewing, otherwise undesirable side effects like suppression of vision may develop. Finally, of course, it is crucial for VDT users to be able to see clearly at close distances and to maintain attention on the screen for extended periods.

Poorly developed visual skills can severely limit the ability of a user to process information displayed on the VDT display screen. The VDT user may have to expend extra effort to perform the job which can lead to visual stress symptoms. If an eye examination reveals any deficiencies in visual skills, then visual training exercises can be recommended to improve visual efficiency.

This chapter presents exercises that are useful in improving visual skills and abilities to reduce visual fatigue. These exercises include a sample **vision therapy** (visual training) program recommended by behavioral optometrists to maintain vision fitness. For optimal results from visual training, a more detailed, specific program should be personally prescribed by a behavioral optometrist. The basic principles underlying vision therapy are as follows:

1. An individualized program of arranging visual conditions and challenges to teach a person more efficient, highly developed control of visual abilities and skills.
2. A method of teaching someone more comfortable, efficient use of the visual system.
3. A visual rehabilitation program based upon the results of behavioral optometric testing.

4. The uniqueness of behavioral optometric visual training versus occupational training is seen by the use of specialized lenses and prisms to change and effect visual spatial processing of information.

VISUAL TRAINING EXERCISES

Some important exercises for visual training are listed below. The emphasized visual skill is in parenthesis following the exercise name. Most of the exercises utilize more than one visual skill at a time.

It is worth emphasizing that these home or work based visual training exercises are useful as a general way to enhance visual skills and abilities necessary for comfort and efficiency while working with VDTs. The disadvantage of this generic approach to visual training is the unavailability of professional optometric consultation concerning variations in technique, timing, styles of training, and scheduling. In addition, a doctor of optometry can include more specific visual training activities which may be of greater benefit for maximum improvement of your visual abilities.

An outline of a visual training schedule for one week using five procedures is included. This schedule can be used for as many weeks as you desire as a visual training maintenance and enhancement program. Discuss any difficulties or concerns with a doctor of optometry.

The outlined visual fitness training schedule is designed for the VDT worker not currently experiencing visual stress symptoms. These visual fitness exercises are most useful when combined with the appropriate stress relieving prescription lenses (computer eyeglasses).

Variations of this recommended schedule can be discussed with your doctor of optometry.

Day 1	Palming, Calendar-Book Rock, Brock String
Day 2	Palming, Thumb Rotations, Form Field Card
Day 3	Palming, Calendar-Book Rock, Thumb Rotations
Day 4	Palming, Brock String, Form Field Card
Day 5	Palming, Calendar-Book Rock, Form Field Card
Day 6	Palming, Brock String, Thumb Rotations
Day 7	Palming, Thumb Rotation, Calendar-Book Rock

This training schedule should be combined daily with physical stretching exercises at your workstation (stretching exercises are discussed later in this chapter).

Palming (Visualization)

Purpose: This important technique will relax your visual system and help neutralize stress, eyestrain, and headaches.

You can do it at a table or your desk, while seated in your chair. Since the goal is relaxation, you may find it helpful to support your arms with cushions or pillows. If you work in an office, support your arms on a typewriter or a pile of telephone directories.

Key Procedure: First, rub your hands together to warm them. Close you eyes and cover them with cupped hands so that no light gets in. (Figure 15). Rest the heel of your palms on your cheekbones and cross your hands on your forehead. Do not apply any pressure to the eyes themselves, and make sure that the eyelids, eyebrows, and fingers are relaxed.

Now breathe slowly and deeply. Relax, and imagine that you are on a tropical beach. It is a warm beautiful day, and you don't have a care in the world. The surf is gently breaking, and you can see the palm trees swaying in the

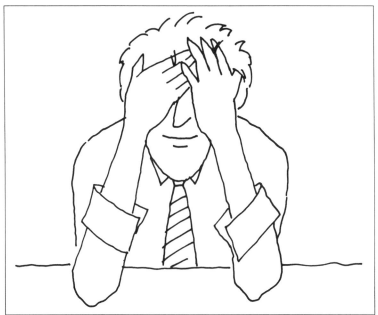

Figure 15. Position for Palming Exercise

breeze. Enjoy the fantasy and visualize as much detail as you can. **Note:** You should select your own fantasy setting. Keep in mind that the ideal visualization is of a wide open setting (ocean, mountain, etc). **Time:** One to five minutes without stopping. Repeat throughout the day for a relaxing break

Calendar - Book Rock (Focusing)

Purpose: To develop rapid and accurate shifts in focusing and localization between near and far areas while processing information.

Materials: Calendar or letter chart. Book, magazine, or other reading material.

Method:

1. Place a calendar or letter chart far enough across the room, so that the numbers (letters) on it are just readable (see Figure 16).
2. The reading material should be held or propped at the reading level and distance (about 15 inches).
3. Read the first 3 numbers (or letters if a letter chart is used) on the top line of the calendar across the room, as quickly as possible. Then read the first sentence or line of the reading material. Continue to repeat the exercise, viewing the next 3 numbers on the calendar and next line of the reading material.
4. Once the print is cleared at near and far easily and quickly, gradually move the near target in to six inches from the eyes. Then see how quickly the letters on the chart can be cleared.

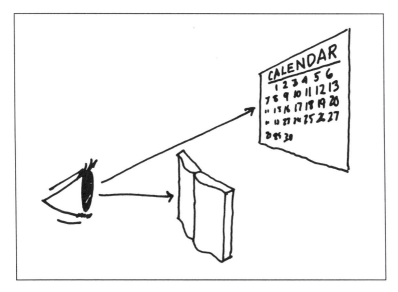

Figure 16. Calendar - Book Rock Diagram

5. Vary the calendar instructions. For example, read the first 4 or 5 numbers. If necessary start with only 2 numbers. Or, read numbers I, 2, 3, or 4 of each line starting with the final number and reading to the left, or starting with the correct internal number, reading to the right.

Emphasized Areas:
1. Ability to keep place close up and on the calendar.
2. Ability to clear the far and near print immediately with change of fixation.
3. Use both eyes together and your prescription eyeglasses if normally worn for distance and near viewing.
Time: 3 - 1 minute cycles per day.

Brock String (Eye Teaming, Focusing)

Purpose: This training procedure teaches the use of both eyes at the same time. It further develops the ability to shift two-eyed vision from one point in space to another point in space easily and quickly without suppressing one eye. The ability to accurately localize in space is also enhanced with this technique.

Materials: An eight foot piece of string with a colored bead at a distance of thirteen inches from one end.

Method:

1. Fasten the string to a stationary object at eye level. Hold the other end of the string between the thumb and forefinger against your nose. The colored bead on the string should be at 10 inches from your eyes and the end of the string should be at some object 8 feet away. Stretch the string tightly so that it extends from the nose to its fastened end in a straight line (see Figure 17).

2. Look at the end of the string and you should see two strings emerging from the side of your head and meeting in a "V" at the fastened end. This is the normal response.

3. If only one string is seen, then this indicates suppression or non-use of one eye. In order to see two strings the following procedure must be followed. Take your hand and cover one eye. Shift your hand from one eye to the other. Every once in awhile look for the "V" with both eyes open.

4. When a "V" can be seen, look at the "V" and then look at the colored bead. You should now see an "X" meeting at the bead and continuing through the bead.
5. As improvement occurs, place another colored bead on the string half way between the other bead, and look from one to the other every five seconds.

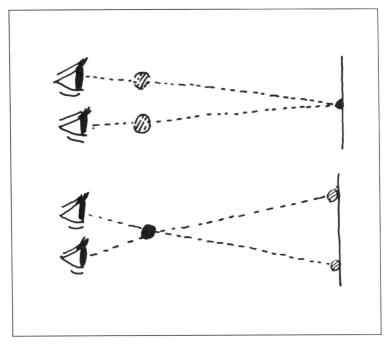

Figure 17. Brock String Diagram

The string should always cross at the bead where you are looking and should appear as an "X".
6. As training proceeds the length of the string may be increased from 8 feet to 12 feet and several different colored beads may be added. This will

induce further divergence of the eyes.

7. Repeat the above procedures, with head turned up, down, left, and right. Note and record location of any areas of suppression (disappearance of string or beads).

8. Use prescription eyeglasses if normally worn for distances described in above instructions.

Time: 3 - 1 minute cycles per day.

Thumb Rotations (Eye Movement)

Purpose: To improve eye movement control and the ability to organize visual space.

Materials: Your own left or right thumb. Wear eyeglasses if normally worn for close working tasks.

Method:

1. Stand erect in a relaxed posture.

2. One eye is covered with the hand on the same side (see Figure 18).

3. The other hand is held out directly in front of the nose, elbow straight, fingers gently clenched, and thumb erect. This point is called the starting point.

4. Look at your thumbnail.

5. Begin to move your arm up, then outward and downward to a point that is level with the nose. Then move it to the starting point again. The thumb should have moved in an outline of a quarter circle.

6. Continue to follow your thumbnail with your eye while your arm traverses the route smoothly and easily.

7. Repeat six times in each direction.

8. Move only your arm and eyeball.

9. Do not pause at any of the reference points mentioned.
10. Repeat for other eye.
11. As this activity is continued, increase your awareness of objects in the room around you.

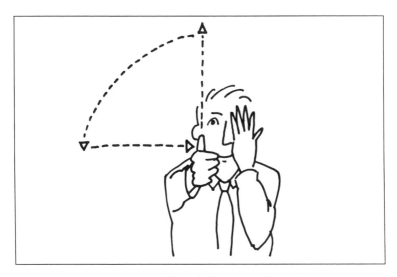

Figure 18. Thumb Rotations Exercise

Emphasized Areas:
1. Ability to follow thumb easily, smoothly with no strain, while the rest of the body remains in an erect, relaxed posture.
2. Thumbnail should remain clear.
   Time: Perform this procedure for two minutes daily with each eye.

Macdonald Form Field Card
(Peripheral Awareness)

Material: Form Field Card (see Figure 19)
Method:
1. Hold card at about 16 inches from eyes
2. Maintain steady fixation on center point of card.
3. While looking only at the card center, observe and record as many letters as possible in the four oblique angles of the card.
4. Use prescription glasses only if necessary to maintain clear focus on central fixation point.

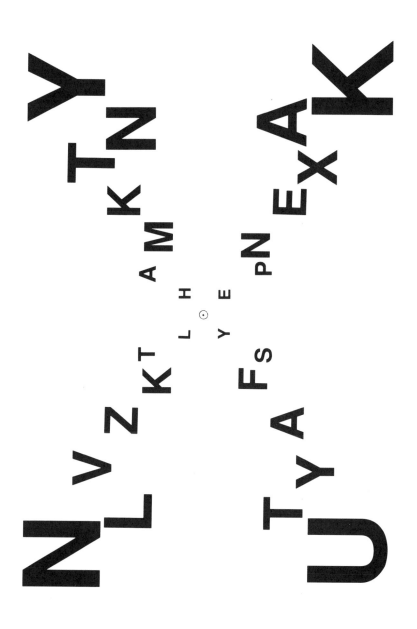

STRETCHING EXERCISES

Basic stretching exercises are also useful in helping to release stress and promote relaxation. Stretching exercises can be done while seated at your workstation and are not strenuous enough to cause you to work up a sweat. It only takes a few minutes to run through the series of exercises listed below and you will feel refreshed. Except where noted otherwise, **repeat each exercise 3 to 5 times.**

Reach for the Sky (arms, shoulders)

1. Raise your arms straight overhead and take a deep breath.
2. Stretch the arms as high as they will go and hold for a count of three.
3. Slowly lower the arms down, while exhaling.

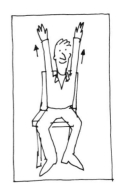

Flower Picking (abdominals, arms)

1. Slide out to the edge of your seat.
2. Bend at the waist and lower your arms (towards the flower bed).
3. Try to touch the floor with your hands.

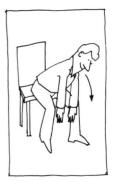

4. Stretch and imagine you are reaching for a beautiful flower.

The Lighthouse (neck, upper back)

1. Pretend you are the lighthouse and your beam is slowly sweeping the horizon.
2. Clasp your hands behind your neck while facing forward.
3. Turn to the right, stretch comfortably, and hold for a count of three.
4. Return so you are facing forward again.
5. Now, turn to the left, stretch comfortably again, and hold for a count of three.
6. Return to the start position.

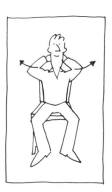

Priming the Pump (legs, thighs)

1. Visualize an old hand pump out on the back porch of a farmhouse.
2. Slide your chair back from your desk to give your legs room.
3. Clasp you hands together just beneath your right knee.

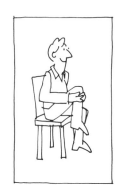

4. Now slowly raise your right leg
   off the floor as you pull back with your arms.
5. Continue to pull back with the arms and lift the legs
   higher off the floor. Develop a good stretch
   in the leg muscles and count to three.
6. Slowly lower the leg back to the floor.
7. Now "prime the pump" using your left leg this time.

Hoisting the Mainsail (arms, shoulders, back)

1. Clasp you hands together behind the back of your
   chair (arms should extend over the top of the chair).
2. Slowly move your hands
   downward and outward
   away from your back.
3. Develop a good stretch
   as you pretend your
   raising the mainsail.
4. Arch the your shoulders
   back and imagine the
   sail filling with wind.
5. Hold for a count of three
   and then relax.

Flipping Flapjacks (hands, wrists)

1. Its a lazy Sunday morning and time to make
   some flapjacks for breakfast.
2. Sit upright with arms bent at elbow. Hold the
   lower part of the arm parallel to the floor.
3. Open and close the hands as you imagine
   mixing the flapjack batter. Repeat 5 times.

4. Now its time to cook
up a stack of flapjacks.
Open your hands with
palms facing down.
Quickly, flip the flapjack
by turning your palms up.
5. Turn your palms down to
place another flapjack on
the griddle. Palms up to
flip another flapjack.

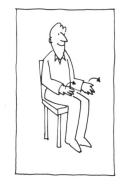

Repeat 5 times (unless you have a bigger appetite).
Steps 3 through 5 should be repeated 3 times.

Our sense of sight should not be isolated from the rest of our being. If we feel good and are healthy, then our work productivity increases. We also enjoy leisure time much more. Because of this it is important to take part in some physical activities each week, particularly if we have a sedentary job.

The activity can be bicycling, chopping wood, swimming, square dancing, or whatever. Preferably the activity should be one that you enjoy. Remember we are not designed for a sedentary existence. Our ancestors were hunters and gatherers. Get up and move around. The dividends that a little bit of exercise will pay back are surprising.

Proper nutrition and restful sleep are other obvious health factors that should not be overlooked. You should strive to maintain balance in your personal and work life. The better our conditioning the better we are able to withstand the stress and demands of our fast-paced technological world.

CHAPTER 6 - VDT HEALTH RISKS AND THE INDIVIDUAL

Computers are part of the daily existence of a growing number of Americans. Computers touch our lives in many ways. Airline reservations, banking transactions, telephone directory assistance, and mail order catalog purchases are just a few of the ways computers are streamlining modern life. Each day more people are using computers, either on the job or at home.

Although computers improve our lives, they are not without health risks. Studies have shown that job type and number of hours per day of VDT use are important factors in determining the extent of reported VDT-related problems. Eye problems are the most common complaints cited by computer users.

This book describes how visual stress results from computer use. Part of the problem results from the inadequacy of our visual systems to handle the demands of VDT use. Only recently have we had to rely so heavily on our eyes for close-up use for extended periods. The other part of the problem relates to poorly designed work environments. Inadequate attention to workstation placement and design leads to eye problems.

In addition to visual complaints there are other areas of health concerns related to computer use. Three other major areas of identified health risks are (1) musculoskeletal problems, (2) stress, and (3) radiation-related effects. We have discussed how stress and musculo-skeletal problems relate to visual stress. However, stress and musculo-skeletal complaints are problem areas in their own right. Reproductive disorders, skin rashes, cataracts, and epileptic reactions have all been cited as possible radiation-related effects of VDT use. These topics all deserve more thorough coverage, but are beyond the scope this book.

Reproductive disorders are of particular concern. Clusters of birth defects and miscarriages have been reported among VDT users in Canada and the United States.[25,26] Research is being conducted to determine if VDT use causes birth disorders. Until more definitive results are available, it would be wise for pregnant women to try to reduce or eliminate time spent using a computer terminal.

So what is the solution to the health risks associated with computer use? There is no simple solution. Action can be taken in several areas including research, education, and legislation.

At present more scientific study is needed to isolate and assess how factors related to the VDT and its use can affect our health. Many existing studies, because of poor design, suffer from lack of conclusive findings.

Education of the public, especially computer users, can play a key role in controlling the health risks of computer use. The more you know the better you can judge and protect yourself from the inherent risks associated with computer use. A well informed public can decide about the need for manufacturing standards and legislation required to protect the VDT user.

Ultimately, legislation will provide the guidelines for computer use. Legislation should be formulated based on scientific findings and the requests of an informed public.

The Council on Scientific Affairs of the American Medical Association (AMA) in 1987 published the following recommendations concerning the health effects of VDTs.[27] The Council on Scientific Affairs recommends that:

"1. the National Institute for Occupational Safety and Health and other groups continue investigations into the nature of VDT worker complaints, with emphasis on ergonomics and stress-reduction measures to reduce worker discomforts and to improve the job environment;

2. the American Medical Association encourages corporate management to be more cognizant of the importance of the man-machine interface, to provide a work environment that reflects this cognizance, and to encourage effective communication between system planners and users; and

3. the AMA continue to monitor this field and alert physicians and other responsible parties if adverse health effects appear to be suggested."

The present state of affairs concerning the health risks of computers is jumbled. The absence of conclusive scientific evidence on the adverse effects of VDTs allows both employers and manufacturers to waffle about taking responsibility for worker safety. It is up to you, the VDT user, to become informed and take responsibility for your own well being.

REFERENCES

1. Naisbitt, J., *Megatrends*, Warner Books, New York, NY. 1984, 333 pp.

2. Hawken, P. *The Next Economy*, Ballentine Books, New York, NY. 1983, 242 pp.

3. Kavner, R.S. and L. Dusky, *Total Vision*, A&W Publishers, Inc., New York, NY. 1978, 264 pp.

4,7, National Academy of Science, National Research Council,
18, *Video Displays, Work, and Vision*, National Academy Press,
20. Washington, DC., 1983, 273 pp.

5. Rose, L. "Workplace Video Display Terminals and Visual Fatigue," *J. of Occupational Medicine*, 23(4), 1987, pp. 321-324.

6. DeMatteo, B. *Terminal Shock*, NC Press Limited, Toronto, 1985, 224 pp.

8. Smith, M.J., B.G. Cohen, and L.W. Stammerjohn Jr., "An Investigation of Health Complaints and Job Stress in Video Display Operations," *Human Factors*, 23, 1981, pp. 395-396.

9. Resko, D.R. and P.K. Mansfield, "Video Display Terminals: How they affect the health of clerical workers," *AAOHN Journal*, 35(7), 1987, pp. 310-314.

10, "VDTs and Vision," Santa Ana, CA, Optometric Extension
11. Program Foundation, COMM4/VDTREPORT1, 12 pp., 1985.

12. Leibowitz, H.L. and D.A. Owens, "Anomalous myopia and the intermediate dark focus of accommodation," *Science*, 189, 1975, pp. 646-648.

13. Murch, G. "How Visible is Your Display?" *Electro-Optical Systems Design*, 14(3), 1982, pp. 43-49.

14. Fahrbach, P.A. and L.J. Chapman, "VDT Work Duration and Musculoskeletal Discomfort," *AAOHN Journal*, 38(1), 1990, pp. 32-36.

15. Starr, S.J, Shute, S.J,, and C.R. Thompson, "Relating Posture to Discomfort in VDT Use," *J. of Occupational Medicine*, 27(4), 1985, pp. 269-271.

16. Pierce, J.R. "Research on the Relationship Between Nearpoint Lenses, Human Performance, and Physiological Activity of the Body," Optometric Extension Program Courses, *Research Reports and Special Articles*, 39(1-12), 1966-1967.

17. World Health Organization, "Work with Visual Display Terminals: Psychosocial Aspects and Health," *J. of Occupational Medicine*, 31(2), 1989, pp. 957-968.

19. Billete, A. and J. Piche, "Health Problems of Data Entry Clerks and Related Job Stressors," *J. of Occupational Medicine*, 29(12), 1987, pp. 942-948.

21. Westin, A.F., H.A. Schweder, M.A. Baker, and S. Lehman. *The Changing Workplace: A Guide to Managing the People, Organizational and Regulatory Aspects of Office Technology*, Knowledge Industry Publications, White Plains, NY, 1985.

22, Margach, C.B., "Video Display Terminals - I,"
23. Santa Ana, CA, Optometric Extension Program
Curriculum II, *Literature & Research Review*, Vol. 60 (6),
March 1988.

24 "Study, Special Glasses Relieve VDT Strain," *Review of
Optometry*, Feb, 1988, p. 8.

25. Goldhaber, M.K., M.R. Polen, and R.A. Hiatt, "The Risk of
Miscarriage and Birth-Defects Among Women Who Use
Visual-Display Terminals During Pregnancy,"
Am. J. of Industrial Medicine, 13(6), 1988, pp. 695-706.

26. McDonald, A.D., N.C. Cherry, C. Delorme, and J.C.
McDonald, "Visual Display Units and Pregnancy: Evidence
From the Montreal Survey," *J. of Occupational Medicine*,
28(12), 1986, pp. 1226-1231.

27 American Medical Association, Council on Scientific Affairs,
"Health Effects of Video Display Terminals," *JAMA*, Vol. 257,
No. 11, March, 1987, pp. 1506-1512.

GLOSSARY

Accommodation (visual)
Eye focusing ability of the eyes.
Acuity (visual)
A measure of the ability of the eye to resolve fine detail.
Astigmatism
An eye defect which causes imperfect focusing.
Awareness - A conscious ability to focus energy and attention.
Behavioral Optometry
A branch of optometry based on an behavioral model of vision. This model states that vision can be trained and enhanced. Behavioral optometry is a holistic approach to visual health and includes "functional" and "developmental" optometry.
Binocularity
Using both eyes as a team to track information or focus on an object.
Bug
An error in a computer program.
Cataracts
Opacity of the lens or capsule of the eye which causes partial or total blindness.
Cathode Ray Tube (CRT)
A glass tube that forms part of most video display terminals. The tube generates a stream of electrons that strike the phosphor coated display screen and cause light to be emitted. The light forms characters on the screen.

Console
Another name for a Computer Terminal or Video Display Terminal.

Convergence
Bringing the eyes together a close range to focus on a particular point of interest.

Cursor
A symbol, usually either a flashing block or dash, that indicates the current input position on the VDT screen.

Digitizer
A computer input device that converts analog signals to digital form. A digitizing pad has a special pen that traces lines or plots separate points creating digital data that are input to the computer.

Diplopia
Term for double vision, which results from the breakdown of eye coordination skills.

Dot Matrix
A pattern of dots that forms characters (text) or constructs a display image (graphics) on the VDT screen.

Electro-static Charge
A form of static electricity. An electro-static charge results from a difference between the negative and positive charges on two objects.

Electromagnetic Radiation
A form of energy resulting from electric and magnetic effects which travels as invisible waves.

Ergonomics
Study of the relationship between humans and their work. The goal of ergonomics is to increase worker comfort, productivity and safety.

Eyestrain (asthenopia)
Descriptive term for symptoms of visual discomfort. Symptoms include burning, itching, tiredness, aching, soreness, and watering.

Farsightedness
A visual condition where objects at distance are more easily focused, as opposed to objects up close.

Font
A complete set of characters (letters, numbers, punctuation, and symbols) including typeface, style, and size used for screen or printer displays.

Focal Length
The distance from the eye to the viewed object needed to obtain clear focus.

Hertz (Hz)
Cycles per second. Used to express the refresh rate of VDTs.

Holistic
An attempt is to see the whole situation and to be careful not to diagnose or treat only parts of the total human performance system.

Lag
In optometric terms, the measured difference between the viewed object and the actual focusing distance.

Luminance
A measure of the brightness of a surface. Luminance is used to describe the brightness of characters on the VDT screen.

Mouse
A computer input device connected by cable to the VDT. The mouse is moved by hand to position the

cursor on the VDT screen. Two or three buttons on the mouse provide a means of selecting screen options.

Myopia (nearsightedness)
Technical term for nearsightedness. The ability to see objects clearly only at a close distance.

Musculo-skeletal
Relating to the muscles and skeleton of the human body.

Nearpoint (near vision)
Relating to close-up vision.

Nearsightedness
See myopia.

Neurology
Study of or relating to the nervous system.

Normal Polarity (normal video)
Computer screen display with light characters against a dark background; analogous to a photographic negative.

Ocular Motility
Eye movement skills.

Perception
Understanding of sensory input (vision, hearing, touch, smell, and/or taste).

Pixel
The smallest element of a display screen that can be independently assigned color and intensity.

Phosphor
A substance that emits light when stimulated by electrons.

Presbyopia
Reduction in the ability to focus on near objects caused by the decreased flexibility of the lens in individuals

usually older than 40.

Resting Point of Accommodation (RPA)
The point in space where the eyes naturally focus when at rest.

Reverse Polarity (reverse video)
Screen display with dark characters against a light background; analogous to printed page.

Refractive
Having the ability to bend light to provide sharp optical imagery.

Refresh Rate
The number of times per second that the screen phosphor must be painted to maintain proper character display.

Scrolling
The movement of information onto and off of the display screen in a vertical manner. Generally new information moves onto the screen at the top and departs at the bottom. Scrolling can occur line by line or by an entire screen full of information.

Suppression
In clinical terms, the "turning off" of the visual functioning of an eye.

Swim
A wave-like motion of screen display information, usually in a vertical direction, due to electrical malfunctioning in the VDT.

Video Display Terminal (VDT)
An electronic device consisting of a monitor unit (e.g., cathode ray tube), connection to a computer central processing unit, and input device (e.g., keyboard).

VDT
Abbreviation for Video Display Terminal.

Vision
A learned awareness and perception of visual experiences (combined with any or all other senses) that results in mental/or physical action.

Visual Stress
Inability of a person to visually process light information in a comfortable, efficient manner.

Visual Training (vision therapy)
Behavioral optometric treatment method used to develop and enhance visual abilities. Visual training consists of eye training procedures.

Visualization
A sophisticated visual skill of using the "mind's eye" to understand visual information.

Workstation
(1) Equipment used by a computer operator, usually consisting of keyboard, computer, and display terminal; (2) A station where a computer operator can send data to or receive data from a computer to perform a particular task.

INFORMATION SOURCES

The following is an listing of additional sources of information about health issues related to VDT use. The listing is by no means comprehensive. Consult your local, state, and regional health and labor organizations for additional information.

The authors encourage reader comments or suggestions about this book. Readers who are CompuServe members may contact the authors by electronic mail.

Dr. Edward Godnig
11 Shapleigh Road
Kittery, Maine 03904
CompuServe User ID number 72557,1135

John Hacunda
P.O. Box 145
Kenyon, RI 02836
CompuServe User ID number 76446,474

VISION RELATED

American Academy of Optometry
5530 Wisconsin Ave., N.W.
Suite 1149
Washington, DC 20815
(301) 652-0905

American Optometric Association (AOA)
243 North Lindbergh Blvd.
St. Louis, MO 63141
(314) 991-4100

Better Vision Institute
220 Park Ave.
New York, NY 10160
(212) 682-1731

National Association of Optometrists and Opticians
18903 South Miles Rd.
Cleveland, OH 44128
(216) 475-8925

Optometric Extension Program Foundation, Inc. (OEP)
2912 South Daimler
Santa Ana, CA 92705
(714) 250-8070

The College of Optometrists in Vision Development (COVD)
P.O. Box 285
Chula Vista, CA 92012-0285
(619) 425-6191

HEALTH RELATED

American Council on Science and Health
1995 Broadway, 18th floor
New York, NY 10023
(212) 362-7044

American Public Health Association
1015 15th St. NW
Washington, DC 20005
(202) 789-5600

Council on Scientific Affairs
American Medical Association
535 North Dearborn St.
Chicago, IL 60610

Industrial Health Foundation
34 Penn Circle West
Pittsburgh, PA 15206
(412) 363-6600

National Health Council
622 3rd Ave., 34th floor
New York, NY 10017-6765
(212) 972-2700

National Safety Council
444 North Michigan Ave.
Chicago, IL 60611
(312) 527-4800

National Wellness Association
Univ. of Wisconsin Stevens Point
South Hall
Stevens Point, WI 54481
(715) 346-2172

National Institute of Occupational Safety and Health (NIOSH)
4676 Columbia Parkway
Cincinnati, OH 45226
(513) 533-8236, (800)-35-NIOSH

Occupational Safety and Health Administration (OSHA)
U.S. Department of Labor
200 Constitution Avenue NW
Washington, DC 20216
(800) 282-1048

Society for Occupational and Environmental Health
P.O. Box 42360
Washington, DC 20015-0360
(202) 762-9319

VDT News
P.O. Box 1799, Grand Central Station,
New York, NY 10163
(212) 517-2802

The Wellness Councils of America
1823 Garbet Street, Suite 201
Omaha, Nebraska 68102
(402) 444-1711

LABOR RELATED

9 to 5, National Association of Working Women
614 Superior Avenue NW
Cleveland, OH 44113
(216) 566-1699, (800) 245-9865

Center for Office Technology
575 Eighth Avenue, 14th Floor,
New York, NY 10018
(21) 560-1298

Massachusetts Coalition on New Office Technology (CNOT)
241 St. Botolph St.
Boston, MA 02107
(617) 536-TECH

Office Technology Education Project
Massachusetts Division of Occupational Hygiene
6 Newsome Park
Jamaica Plain, MA 02130
(617) 524-4040

SAMPLE QUESTIONNAIRE TO DISCUSS WITH YOUR VISION CARE PROFESSIONAL

WORK PRACTICES

1. Number of hours per workday of VDT viewing? _____
2. If # 1 is more than 2 hours, what rest periods, (duration, number) do you have? _____
3. Check whether your work at the VDT is varied _____, or is not varied _____
4. If you have regular rest breaks, describe what you do during those breaks. Is a "visual relief" area provided? _____
   _____
   _____
5. How long have you been working on this VDT viewing job? ___
6. How frequently does a video technician do routine maintenance on your VDT unit? _____
7. How often is your VDT screen cleaned? _____
   By whom? _____

ROOM ENVIRONMENT

8. As you sit facing your VDT screen, what bright sources of light can you see as you look straight ahead? List them, including uncurtained windows and unshielded overhead lighting:
   _____
   _____
9. Using a hand mirror held parallel and adjacent to the screen, what objects on your side of the screen (including yourself) can you see reflected in it?
   _____
   _____
10. Do the walls of your VDT viewing room have shiny _____ or dull _____ surfaces?
11. What color are the walls of your room? _____

12. Overall, how bright is your viewing room as compared with the brightness in most office workrooms? About the same ___, half as bright ____, twice as bright ____, other:_____
13. How noisy is your viewing room, as compared with a room full of typist? About the same ____, more noisy ____, less noisy ____
14. How comfortable is the room temperature? Too hot ____, too cold ____, just right ____, drafty ____, air conditioned____
15. How is the air quality? Smoky ____, stale ____, dry ____, humid ____

SCREEN

16. What color is the screen background? _____
    Reversible polarity possible? Yes ____ No ____
17. What colors are the characters?_____
18. Is the brightness of the background adjustable by you? ____
19. Is the brightness of the characters adjustable by you? _____
20. Is the background brightness adjustment independent of the character brightness adjustment? _____
21. Distance of screen from eyes when in usual viewing posture? _____ in. _____ cm.
22. Vertical location of top edge of screen? At eye level ____, above ____, or below ____ eye level, ____ ins. ____ cm ____
23. Characters: If all capitals: Letter M is ____ mm high and ____ mm wide. If upper & lower: Lower case "o" is ____ mm high. Number of characters per line of display ____
    Quality: Sharp ____ Blurred ____ Average____
    Readability: Good ____ Poor ____ Average ____
    New information is added to the screen: One line at a time____, Letter by letter ____, Too fast____, too slow ____, Just right ____ Number of lines of characters when screen is full: _____
24. Can screen tilt be altered by you? Yes____ No ____
25. Does display flicker for you? Yes ____ No ____
26. Does the screen have a hood? Yes ____ No ____
    Glare filter? Yes ____ No ____ Security filter? Yes ____ No ____
27. Color of VDT?_____ Finish: dull ____, shiny ____

28. Cursor: steady _____, blinking _____, either _____
29. Swim: Yes _____ No _____; peripheral distortions: Yes_____
    No _____; error flashes: Yes _____ No _____

WORKSTATION

30. Make and Model of VDT used? _____
31. Supporting surface for VDT adjustable for height? Yes _____
    No _____
32. Supporting surface for console adjustable for height? Yes___
    No _____
33. Supporting surface for copy adjustable for height? Yes _____
    No _____
34. Present viewing distances: eyes to screen _____ in. _____ cm
35. Could copy, console, and screen all be at the same viewing
    distance? Yes _____ No _____
36. Is copy surface large enough to accept largest materials you
    use? Yes _____ No _____
37. Is copy support used? Yes _____ No _____
38. Chair: stable base? Yes _____ No _____
    adjustable seat height? Yes _____ No _____
    adjustable seat area? Yes _____ No _____
    adjustable back support height? Yes _____ No _____
    adjustable back support tension? Yes _____ No _____
    can adjustments be made without tools? Yes _____ No _____
39. Are all working components fully visible without trunk
    movements? Yes _____ No _____
40. Working posture: upper arm angle _____forearm angle _____
    trunk line _____thigh angle _____; thigh support _____
    foot position _____; foot rest _____
41. Copy is: easy to read _____, hard to read _____, varies _____
42. Copy stock is: dull _____, shiny _____, color _____
43. Is auxiliary lighting available? Yes _____ No _____

CONSOLE

44. Is console movable (detached from video screen)? Yes _____
    No_____

45. Angle of wrist when operating keyboard: _____
46. Console keyboard: flat _____, inclined _____, adjustable _____
47. Palm rest? Yes _____ No _____
48. Feedback from operation of keyboard: audible _____,
    tactile_____
49. Keytops recessed? Yes _____ No _____
50. Readability of keytops: difficult _____, easy _____,
    average_____
51. Color of keytops: _____
52. Color of characters on keys: _____
53. Reflections: keytops _____, console _____

JOB RELATED VISUAL QUESTIONS

54. Do you have eyestrain or visual fatigue that occurs on the
    job? Yes _____ No _____
55. If you answer "yes" to # 54 above, describe what happens:
    a. Headaches? Yes _____ No _____ When? _____
       How long? _____ Stopped by? _____
    b. Blurring of nearby objects like your watch dial? Yes_____
       No _____
    c. Blurring of distant objects across the room, or on your way
       home? Yes _____ No _____
    d. Blurring of letters on screen? Yes _____ No _____
       When?____ Stopped by? _____
56. Do you have bodily discomfort, such as neck, shoulder, or
    wrist pain? Yes _____ No _____
    a. If "yes," describe type of discomfort? _____
    b. If "yes," when does it occur? _____
    c. If "yes," how long does it last? _____
    d. If "yes," does it improve during breaks? _____
57. Does your error rate change during the day? Yes _____
    No_____
    a. If "yes," describe how it changes: _____
    b. If "yes," is it tied in with questions # 54, # 55, and or# 56?
    Describe:_____
    _____

(Reprinted with permission. OEP Foundation, Santa Ana, CA)

58. Describe your general reactions to your VDT viewing job, as compared with more conventional jobs. (Suggestions: rewarding exciting, challenging, frustrating, fatiguing, dull, etc.)

_____

_____

_____

ABOUT THE AUTHORS

Edward C. Godnig, O.D., is a graduate of the New England College of Optometry, Boston, Massachusetts. He is in private practice in Kittery, Maine, specializing in behavioral optometry. Dr. Godnig is a Fellow of the College of Optometrists in Vision Development, a full scope optometric care organization dedicated to the enhancement of vision. He is also a Clinical Associate of the Optometric Extension Program, an international continuing education and research organization dedicated to advance progress through education in behavioral vision care. Dr. Godnig's other interests include alpine and cross country skiing, bicycle touring, hiking in the White Mountains, and Cub Scout leadership activities.

John S. Hacunda, M.S. has experience as a biologist, software engineer, and technical writer. Mr. Hacunda has designed and developed software for sound/speech synthesis applications and telecommunications systems. He is a Member of the Institute of Electrical and Electronic Engineers and a Corporation Member of the Bermuda Biological Station for Research. He enjoys outdoor activities and has sailed to the Galapagos Islands.

ORDER FORM

Seacoast Information Services
4446 South County Trail
Charlestown, RI 02813

Please send me ___ copy(s) at $8.95 each of

COMPUTERS and VISUAL STRESS
by
Dr. Edward Godnig and John Hacunda

I understand that if I am not fully satisfied with the book I may return it for a full refund within 30 days.

Name:_____

Address:_____

_____ZIP:_____

Rhode Island Residents: Please add 6% Sales Tax

Shipping: Please add $1 for the first book and 50 cents for each additional book.